Siimon Reynolds is a dir
Anti-Aging Clinic, Austr
specialising in longevity.

Siimon also runs Moon Corporation, an
organisation with major interests in advertising,
gaming, education and technology companies.

Other books by Siimon Reynolds in Pan:

When They Zig You Zag
Become Happy in Eight Minutes

100
ways
to live to
100

Siimon Reynolds

PAN
Pan Macmillan Australia

Acknowledgement is due to Crown Publishers Inc. for permission to quote from
Ageless Body, Timeless Mind © Deepak Chopra.

Acknowledgement is due to Prentice Hall Direct, Division of P.L. Publishing Inc.
for permission to quote from
Look Ten Years Younger, Live Ten Years Longer: A Man's Guide
by David Ryback copyright © 1995.

The information contained in this book is intended to be a general guide for people seeking
to improve their health and longevity. The author and publisher assume no responsibility,
and recommend that you should only follow guidelines contained in this book under
your doctor's supervision.

First published 1999 in Macmillan by Pan Macmillan Australia Pty Limited
St Martins Tower, 31 Market Street, Sydney

Copyright © Siimon Reynolds 1999

National Library of Australia
cataloguing-in-publication data:

Reynolds, Siimon.
100 ways to live to 100.

ISBN 0 330 36178 3.

1. Aging – Prevention. 2. Longevity. I. Title.
II. Title : One hundred ways to live to 100.

613

Typeset in 12/17 pt Avenir Book by Post Pre-Press Group
Printed in Australia by McPherson's Printing Group

To Brian,
a true pioneer of
anti-aging medicine

Contents

Why do some people live longer than others?

Is it just good genes, or is there more to it?

Although only a decade old, anti-aging medicine is one of the fastest growing areas of healthcare in the world.

Introduction

Once we thought a long, healthy life was in the lap of the gods; however, we now know there are specific things we can do to slow down and even reverse the aging process.

I've collected the best of these methods in one short, sharp, easy to understand book.

100 Ways To Live To 100 is a summary of the hundreds of hours I have spent studying this subject via mountains of books and scores of lectures and interviews with the world's top anti-aging specialists.

The book also features many of the techniques we utilise at the Redwood Anti-Aging Clinic, Australia's first and largest anti-aging medical centre.

Put this book into practice and you're not only likely to live longer, but the days you live will be filled with energy, vitality and optimism.

Sound great?

Well then, let's get started . . .

100
ways
to live to
100

I

Choose to be happy

Psycho-neuroimmunology sounds a mouthful, but it is one of the most exciting fields of medicine today. Basically it shows that a happy attitude leads to less bodily stress and a boosted immune system.

If you doubt the power of the mind on the body, consider this: more heart attacks happen around 9 a.m. on Monday morning than at any other time! Laughter also radically affects the immune system, increasing the number of T cells, B cells and immunoglobulins.

2

Reduce red meat

Red meat is usually high in fat and often contains poisons. It's also much harder for your stomach to digest than fruit and vegetables.

What's more, according to Dr John Berg's research at the National Cancer Institute, your chances of getting colon cancer increase when you have a high meat intake. Best to play it safe and keep meat to a minimum.

3

Develop a sense of purpose

According to world-renowned longevity expert Dr Vincent Giampapa, people who have a sense of purpose tend to age more slowly than others.

That purpose may come from their work, their family, their spiritual practices or their lifestyle, but having a clear direction and reason to get up in the morning seems to positively affect both stress levels and immunity.

4

Reduce free radicals

Many experts believe free radicals are the number one cause of premature aging. Free radicals are biochemical compounds, produced as a result of toxicity in the body, which damage our cells.

One of the best ways of reducing them is to live a relaxed life and to take the three popular anti-oxidants, vitamins C, B and beta-carotene, daily.

5

Forget frozen
vegetables

According to Ronald Klatz, the President of the American Academy of Anti-Aging Medicine, frozen vegetables aren't nearly as healthy as fresh ones.

In fact, they have around 25 per cent less of the common vitamins like A, C, B1, B2 and B3 than cooked fresh vegetables.

Canned vegies are even worse, possessing two to three times fewer vitamins than frozen vegetables. According to Dr Klatz most canned peas, for example, have lost 96 per cent of their vitamin C content.

6

The soybean miracle

The soybean is one of nature's great anti-aging pills. These little beans are famous amongst nutritionists for their apparent ability to help prevent free radical damage to our cells.

For instance, the Japanese consume 30 times more soy than Americans, and have significantly fewer cases of heart disease, diabetes, cancer and osteoporosis.

Dr Denham Harmon also showed that lab animals that consumed soybean protein enjoyed a 13 per cent longer life.

7

Try the
Mediterranean diet

A study reported in the *British Medical Journal* showed that the typical Mediterranean farmer's diet (rich in olive oil and with small amounts of wine) may increase your life span.

A six-year study of Greek farmers and their wives over 70 years of age showed that those who consumed a diet including olive oil, wholegrain breads, fresh fruit and vegetables 'significantly reduced their chances of dying during the study, compared to those who ate diets rich in red meats and saturated fats'.

8

Fibre power

Fibre can be an excellent weapon in your anti-aging arsenal.

A high-fibre diet reduces your risk of bowel cancer, varicose veins and haemorrhoids. It's also great for your digestion.

Finally, fibre is excellent in helping to lower cholesterol; it acts like a blotter in the intestines.

You can get your fibre intake from broccoli, green lettuce and green beans, and of course, from cereals.

9

Don't get angry

Anger is one of the world's biggest health risks, wreaking havoc on your body's defence system.

Harvard Medical School interviewed 1623 heart attack victims four days after they were hospitalised and found that episodes of anger doubled their risk of heart attack, and that many had suffered the attack just two hours after their anger outburst.

Next time you're angry, leave the room and do some deep breathing to release your body's muscular and mental stress.

10

Say so long to salt

Not only does salt lead to hardening of the arteries, a high salt intake could lead to blood pressure problems.

Give salt a miss whenever you can.

And be sure to watch out for hidden salt. Usually foods that are processed – like canned soup, tomato sauce, luncheon meats and mustard – are also high in salt.

11

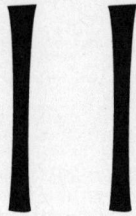

Drink lots of pure water

Most people don't drink nearly enough water. The US National Research Council's recommended daily allowance for water is a quart-and-a-half (nearly one-and-a-half litres) each day.

Any less than this and not only will your skin look older but your kidneys will be less effective as toxin filters.

Don't drink tap water either; it often contains chemicals such as chlorine and fluoride.

12

Go easy on the coffee

More than two cups a day wreaks havoc on your body's nervous system. It increases gastric acid and acts as a diuretic, furthering your fluid loss. There's also some evidence that coffee builds up serum cholesterol levels and the risk of heart trouble.

Swap your coffee for fruit juices or even green tea, which is believed to be a potent anti-cancer beverage.

Get involved

Gerontologists believe that people who really engage in life usually live longer than others.

This concept was first described over 30 years ago by Cumming and Henry in their book *Growing Older*. They noticed that as people grow older they tend to lose contact with others. This disengagement leads to a reduction in physical and mental activity and subsequently a faster rate of body and mind aging.

So get out there and get into life! It's not just more fun, it's actually keeping you alive.

14

Take shark cartilage
tablets

Since the mid 1970s, shark cartilage has been used by cutting-edge doctors to reduce tumours in patients. Cuban and Japanese research studies have found shark cartilage can be a highly successful treatment for many different types of cancer.

Taken by healthy people once or twice a week, it could help prevent this dreaded disease occurring. (Check out the breakthrough book, *Sharks Don't Get Cancer* by Dr William Lane.)

15

Take a mineral
supplement

The US Department of Agriculture discovered that a large percentage of people receive under 70 per cent of the recommended daily allowance of essential minerals (and indeed vitamins).

Most people's diets are desperately short of calcium, magnesium, iron, zinc and copper.

A simple multi-mineral tablet taken once daily can make a huge improvement to your health.

16

Become a vegetarian

The British Medical Association says vegetarians live longer than meat eaters. Vegie scoffers have a 28 per cent lower risk of dying from heart disease and a 39 per cent reduced chance of dying from cancer.

Their findings are the result of a massive 12-year research program involving 5000 British meat eaters and 6100 vegetarians.

17

Boost your fish oils

The oils from fish are called Omega-3 fatty acids and are known to be highly beneficial to health.

In fact, women with a high concentration of Omega-3 fatty acids in their breast tissues are five times less likely to develop deadly tumours than other women.

18

Watch your amino acids

Amino acids are the basic building blocks of the 40,000 different proteins in the body.

Eight amino acids can't be made by the body, so you have to get them from your diet.

See your local health store for a good amino acid supplement or advice on which natural foods are high in these vital nutrients.

19

Think young

Remember that old saying 'You're as young as you feel'?

Recent research suggests it's more than just a common adage.

A Harvard professor took a group of 70-year-olds out to the country for three weeks. There, they were instructed to do chores as if they were young, listen to the same music they listened to when they were youths, read only publications that were current when they were young, and generally act like they were teenagers again.

Subsequent tests revealed they actually showed signs of becoming physically younger, with more energy and better reaction times.

20

Follow supplement
guidelines

Nutritional supplements can greatly aid your health and longevity, but be sure to follow these rules from nutritionists Jeffrey Bland PhD and D Landsey Berkson MA:

- Always take vitamin and mineral supplements with meals to help absorption.
- Always take amino acids on an empty stomach.
- If taking high dosages, spread them out during the day.
- Drink lots of liquid when taking supplements to help digestion and reduce side effects.

21

Have a selenium drink

Many cancer patients are short of the mineral selenium in their diets, according to Gerhard Schrauzer PhD.

Selenium supplements have also slowed or stopped the reappearance of cancer in animals.

You can buy selenium in liquid or powdered form and it's easy to mix it with your morning juices to make a potent health drink.

22

Take CoQ10

It sounds like a scientific formula but CoQ10 is in fact a fantastically potent nutrient for generating energy. But unfortunately, as you get older your body produces less and less of it.

You can get CoQ10 from fish, grapeseed oil, many nuts, spinach and soybeans, or you can take it in capsule form.

The Definitive Guide to Cancer reports that in one study, 90mg of CoQ10 were given to 32 breast cancer patients for two years. All patients survived and six had partial remissions.

23

Have plenty of garlic

For centuries garlic has been used by the Chinese, Japanese and Italians as a medicine and food additive.

Recent studies indicate that garlic has special therapeutic properties that aid longevity.

Research in over 50 universities and institutions has shown that garlic promotes energy, protects against free radicals and reduces stress hormones, according to Lynn Petesch, Kyolic's garlic nutritionist.

24

Ginseng, the ancient wonder

Ginseng has been a favorite of Korean, Japanese and Chinese doctors for over 2000 years.

More recently, a report in *Free Radical Biology and Medicine* stated that ginseng had anti-aging immune enhancements and anti-tumour effects.

When taking ginseng, 500mg a day is usually a good dose for most people.

25

Sleep

Life has got so busy!

The average person has 37 per cent less leisure time than in the 1970s.

Often, this busyness means people cut corners on their sleep, just to save time.

Don't. Research indicates that a shortage of sleep inhibits both the repair of your body and the relaxation of your mind.

Also, try to go to sleep and get up at about the same time each day, to reduce bodily stress even further.

26

Follow Deepak's rules

Dr Deepak Chopra is a legend in the field of mind-body medicine.

In his brilliant book *Ageless Body Timeless Mind* he lists some interesting rules to follow to maximise your longevity.

1. Respond creatively to change.
2. Reduce anxiety.
3. Focus on the ability to create and invent.
4. Maintain high levels of adaptability and flexibility.
5. Integrate new things and ideas into your life.
6. Want to stay alive.

27

Practise yoga

Some of the healthiest old people in the world are the yogis in India.

Indeed longevity is one of the primary reasons Indians practise this ancient art. It not only keeps muscles in shape, it's also said to be wonderful for the nervous system and brain.

For strong physical benefits try Hatha or Iyengar style, and for a more spiritual emphasis try the Raja school.

28

Reduce worry

Worriers seldom live long lives; their nervous system packs up under constant stress.

But how do you stop worrying?

Here is one simple method: change how you view life, from 'It's a war' to 'It's a game'. It can do wonders.

Another technique is to schedule your daily worrying time. For example, say to yourself that you'll do all your worrying from 3 p.m. to 3.30. Try it, it works!

29

Don't diet

Fat people tend to die earlier than slim people, yet diets often make you fatter in the long run. Longevity expert Dr David Ryback explains how this happens:

> **As we lose weight through dieting, fat cells do not shrink in number but merely in size. Once we give up on our diet, those fat cells soak up all the fat they can to regain their normal size and if we continue our fat intake beyond that, then additional fat cells will add to our bulk.**

So dieting starts off well, but then there's a plateau or rebounding effect. It is best just to eat normally, but to only eat low-fat foods.

30

Walk when you can

The more you walk, the less fat you'll have and the better your cardiovascular system will become.

Try these tactics:

- Park your car a few blocks from work or home.
- Always take the stairs.
- Don't eat at the nearest sandwich shop.
- Forget the car for short journeys.

31

Always eat breakfast

Some people think it's healthy to skip breakfast, but the opposite is true.

A good breakfast not only fills you with energy, it also helps your mind process information faster, and reduces bodily stress. Just don't make it a heavy meal. Fruit or muesli with a juice or herbal tea is perfect.

32

Associate with young people

The people around you have a huge impact on your quality of life, and how long you live.

Hang around with young people and you'll act and feel young.

The quality of your support group is also crucial if you get sick.

Dr David Skegel of Stanford University once closely observed two similar groups of cancer patients. Those who participated in weekly support-group sessions not only suffered less pain and anxiety, they also *lived twice as long.*

33

Practise Chi Gung

Thousands of years old, the Chinese art of Chi Gung is now achieving significant growth in the West.

Similar to Tai Chi, Chi Gung has been the subject of countless university research studies in China, and has been found to have a powerful effect on the body's energy levels.

Chi Gung is centered around the theory that in addition to our physical body, humans have an energy body. This energy travels along 'rivers' inside us known as meridians.

The slow, rhythmic movements of Chi Gung help unblock our energy rivers, alleviating stress, disease, and according to many believers, slowing down the aging process. No wonder 60 million Chinese practise it!

A terrific first book for those interested in this mysterious art is *Chi Gung. Cultivating Personal Energy* by James MacRitchie (Element Books).

34

Don't miss out on calcium

Women have long been told to watch their calcium levels, but did you know that the average male needs about 25 per cent more calcium than he gets?

Calcium strengthens bones and is excellent for keeping your blood pressure normal.

Get your calcium fix from low-fat dairy products, fish, fruits and vegetables (especially beans), grains or, of course, calcium supplement pills.

Be careful, though, when taking calcium pills with pills containing iron, as calcium interferes with iron absorption.

35

Magic mushrooms

Longevity experts have long held that mushrooms have potent power.

Consider Shiitake mushrooms, for example. Shiitake contains lentinal, a substance that greatly boosts your T cell production and has been shown to help slow the spread of cancer, particularly of the lungs.

So when you're eating your mushrooms, you're not just eating something tasty, you're actually protecting your life.

36

Good old vitamin C

Yes, we've all known about it for ages, but vitamin C remains one of the great longevity supplements. However, don't go crazy on the doses.

You need between 1 to 3 grams a day, ideally spread out over the day as your body won't store this vitamin. (Should you experience diarrhoea just scale back the dosage.)

What can vitamin C do for you? What doesn't it do! It helps heal wounds, helps prevent cancer, protects against some of the effects of smoking, resists the onset of male infertility and much, much more . . .

37

Zinc puts back the zing

The older we get, the less efficient our immune system becomes.

That's where zinc can help.

Tests on animals show that those short of zinc are more prone to cancer.

Zinc is also great for male sexuality as a shortage of zinc in men has been shown to contribute to a lower sex drive and lower sperm count.

Even arthritis may be helped by taking zinc.

When taking zinc, 25mg a day is a suitable dose for most adults.

38

Watch out for
hotdogs

Those tasty hotdogs could bite your insides to death!

Most hotdogs contain sodium nitrate, which some cancer researchers believe can create carcinogens.

So, stay away from them – even if you're cold and starving at a football game!

39

Fast

The practice of fasting has been common for hundreds of years, and is recommended in such major religions as Christianity, Islam and Buddhism.

This is for a good reason. A one- or two-day fast not only gives your poor old intestines a much-needed break, it also allows them to excrete toxins that may have been stored in your body for months.

An all fruit or vegetable juice fast once or twice a year is a great idea and, if you're particularly keen, a one-day fast each week will do wonders for you.

Obviously, you should discontinue the fast if you feel sick, weak or dizzy . . .

40

Run marathons

In an amazing study, Dr Tom Bassler carried out an ongoing worldwide analysis of mortality amongst marathon runners. His conclusion was that marathon athletes are virtually immune from heart disease, as long as they keep training.

It's a radical theory, but he certainly has some good statistics to back it up.

So if you like going for a jog, lengthening your runs a little (a lot!) may be just the thing for you . . .

41

Check your cosmetics

Many shampoos and lotions contain ingredients believed to be carcinogenic, according to US pharmaceutical expert Thomas Mower PhD.

Read labels carefully and stay away from Sulphur Lauryl Sulfate (SLS) or anything starting with the capital letters PEG. According to Mower, there is some evidence these chemicals may in part be responsible for the growing incidence of Alzheimer's disease in our population.

42

Go slow on fast foods

Excess sodium is bad for you and, unfortunately, most fast food is heavy on sodium. A Big Mac, for instance, has over 200mg of sodium. And let's not even get into how bad french fries are for you!

If you have to eat in a hurry, grab a salad from Pizza Hut or from one of those steak and seafood restaurants, like Sizzler.

43

Don't get too much sun

Your skin gets thinner as you get older, making it more susceptible to the sun's harmful rays.

Your skin cell 'turnover' also begins to slow down in your 30s, meaning that each layer of skin stays longer on your face. (Your skin may look like it's dormant, but it's actually changing all the time.)

Keep your time in direct sunlight down to about half an hour a day. Always use a sunblock, and keep away from the harsh midday sun.

44

Meditate

Testing carried out since 1968 by such respected institutions as Harvard Medical School, Stanford University and New England Hospital clearly shows that daily meditation can dramatically reduce stress and help maintain physical and mental health. Indeed, some of the longest living people in the world are yogis, who are known to be dedicated meditators.

For a proven meditation technique look up Transcendental Meditation in the *Yellow Pages* or order one of Dr Herbert Benson's two great books, *The Relaxation Response* or *Timeless Healing*.

45

Get married

Although it obviously depends on how much plate-throwing goes on, married couples tend to live longer than singles.

Not only that, studies on married people also record that those who have tied the knot generally have greater levels of happiness and life satisfaction than their single counterparts.

Interestingly, Maurine Venters PhD, of the University of Minnesota also reports that separated and divorced people spend longer resting in hospital after a heart attack or stroke.

46

Eat low-fat foods

The world is getting fatter!

It's estimated that a whopping one in three Americans are clinically obese (20 per cent above ideal weight) and Australians are not much better.

This is bad news, as there is overwhelming evidence that a high-fat diet increases the risk of cancer of the colon, breast and prostate.

Excess weight also contributes to many of the diseases of aging including heart disease, stroke and diabetes.

47

Buy organic fruit and vegetables

Are fruit and vegetables good for you?

Not always. Many have been grown with the use of pesticides and even food colouring, some of which could end up in your stomach.

A better bet is to buy only organic fruit and vegetables. Sure, they're a little more expensive, but they're usually much cleaner, purer and more flavour-packed.

48

Follow Heart
Association guidelines

For a long, healthy life it pays to stick to these American Heart Association guidelines.

1. Dietary fat intake should be less than 30 per cent of total calories.
2. Saturated fat should be less than 10 per cent of total fat intake.
3. Carbohydrate intake should represent 50 per cent or more of total calories (with an emphasis on complex carbohydrates).
4. Sodium intake should be less than 3gm per day.

49

Take folic acid daily

Everyone's heard of the vitamins C, B and E, but not many have heard of folic acid. That's a shame, as a report in the journal of the American Medical Association estimated that up to 50,000 deaths from heart disease could be prevented each year if Americans consumed more folic acid.

You can get folic acid by eating leafy vegetables, carrots, egg yolk, pumpkin, beans or as a supplement from your local health food store.

50

Get a pet!

They're not just cute and cuddly, they may also increase your life span.

According to Dr Robert Goldman, co-author of the brilliant anti-aging book *Stopping the Clock*, various studies have shown that pet owners tend to live longer and happier lives than those who don't own a furry friend.

51

Exercise daily

The ultimate longevity technique. Daily vigorous exercise increases the body's production of Human Growth Hormone, which helps regenerate your body's cells. Exercise also reduces stress, which is a crucial factor in aging.

When Harvard University studied 17,000 graduate males aged between 35 and 74, they found that those who exercised had the lowest death rate.

52

Have sex often

It really is the case of use it or lose it!

In his superb book *Dare To Be 100*, Dr Walter Bortz reported that regularly having sex is one of the best ways to keep your sexual organs healthy and strong until old age.

In the case of men, it was also found that regular erections decrease the deposits of collagen, an inhibitor of erections.

53

Be an optimist

Optimistic people tend to get less stressed than pessimists, simply because they tend to believe that everything will be okay and that their problems are temporary rather than permanent. This confident attitude reduces the flow of cortisol (a stress-related hormone) and thus the wear and tear on cells.

Dr Carl Simonton, who has carried out over 20 years of research into what causes and cures cancer, also strongly believes that an optimistic mind can greatly aid health. (See his brilliant book *Getting Well Again*, published by Bantam Books.)

54

Train your brain

Amazingly, your brain can get smarter with your advancing age, not slower. It's all got to do with how much you use it.

Play board games, do crosswords daily, involve yourself socially, read a book a month, play an instrument . . . just participate, and your brain can remain sharp until 100 and beyond.

For more great information on increasing brain power as you get older, read *The Age Conspiracy* by Tony Buzan.

55

Be orderly

According to Walter Bortz, 'When 1200 centenarians were surveyed to find out their secret to longevity, 90 per cent of the group identified the role of order in their lives. Orderliness – not money, not genetics, not health – led the list of beneficial aptitudes'.

So plan your day, plan your year, plan your life. Keep your house clean and your mind clear. Don't rush, don't complicate things, and stick to proven systems.

56

Laugh a lot

Laughter is highly therapeutic.

In fact, Dr Norman Cousins in his classic book *Anatomy of an Illness*, reported curing himself of a rare degenerative disease by watching funny movies for hours each day.

When we laugh, the brain produces 'feel good' chemicals called endorphins, which are believed to improve our immune response.

57

Follow Dr Ryback's anti-cancer diet

A top anti-aging expert and author of *Look Ten Years Younger Live Ten Years Longer*, David Ryback has a five-step plan to prevent the dreaded disease.

1. Help yourself to a serving of wholegrain bread, cereal, pasta or brown rice at least four times a day.
2. Have at least two servings a day of citrus fruits, green peppers or tomatoes.
3. Eat broccoli, cabbage, carrots or cauliflower at least once a day.
4. Enjoy beans or tea a few times a week.
5. Be vegetarian or choose fish or fowl over red meat.

58

Study fire prevention

House fires kill hundreds of people every year, yet a few simple precautions can almost totally eradicate your risk.

Follow these directions for a fire-free life for you and your family:

- Have a smoke alarm installed in your home.
- Purchase a fire blanket and fire extinguisher.
- Keep portable heaters away from combustible materials like curtains, rugs and couches.
- Don't smoke in bed.
- Before you leave the house, check for potential fire hazards: cigarettes still alight, iron and stove still on, etc.

59

Keep three first aid
kits handy

Most families don't even have one first aid kit, but to be really safe you need three:

- One in your house for the numerous home accidents that could be life-threatening (falls, burns, etc).
- One in your workplace, as thousands of people are killed every year by work accidents.
- Finally, one in the boot of your car.

Three kits may cost you a couple of hundred dollars, but surely the increased safety is worth it.

60

Breastfeed your baby

For the longevity of your kids, breastfeeding is far superior to alternative methods.

Indeed, recent evidence suggests that natural breast milk may in fact protect your child from cancer.

The National Institute of Child Health and Human Development in the US found that babies who were breastfed for at least six months had considerably less risk of brain tumours, leukaemia and lymphoma than kids who were fed only formula.

61

Listen to relaxation
tapes

You can buy them at most book or music stores and they can work wonders on your stress levels.

For the best results choose subliminal tapes – they not only have soothing music but are embedded with positive affirmations that enter your subconscious mind.

And relaxation tapes aren't just good for relaxation – classical music (particularly 'Baroque' style) has been proven to increase your ability to learn. (See *Super Learning* by Nancy and Sheila Oestrander for details.)

62

Limit sperm loss

This may seem bizarre advice, but the retention of male sperm is a crucial part of the entire Chinese health system.

Chinese doctors believe a good store of male semen massively boosts the body's immune system and energy levels. According to them, frequent ejaculation prematurely ages males.

For a superb book on this subject check out *The Multi Orgasmic Man* by Mantak Chia and Douglas Abrams Arava (HarperCollins).

63

Limit animal protein

Most of us eat too much animal protein and many of us eat at least 30 per cent too much.

We don't need it. In fact, regularly consuming high amounts of animal protein can be positively harmful – it's often high in saturated fat and cholesterol (which can lead to artery clogging).

So try as much as possible to get your protein from non-animal sources, such as nuts, beans and broccoli.

64

Follow Dr Goldman's anti-depression plan

A depressed life is more likely to be a short life. Longevity specialist Dr Robert Goldman has an eight-step program for beating depression and increasing your good moods.

1. Boost the vitamins B6 and B12 in your diet, along with folic acid and riboflavin.
2. Eliminate sugar and caffeine.
3. Get 30 minutes of sunlight daily and work in very well lit rooms.
4. Eat plenty of complex carbohydrates.
5. Consider taking DLPA.
6. Load up on foods with Omega-3 fatty acids (like fish).
7. Try St Johns Wort.
8. Exercise vigorously three times a week.

65

The daily siesta

Practised by numerous European nations for thousands of years, the siesta, or brief afternoon nap, has recently been found to aid longevity.

A study by the University of Athens Medical School discovered that those men who napped for 30 minutes a day or more were 30 per cent less likely to have heart problems than those who didn't.

66

Aspirin isn't just for
headaches

It seems that taking an aspirin every other day can have a remarkable effect on your health if you're 50 or older.

Researchers from the Brigham and Warners Hospital in Boston found that taking this common headache pill may reduce the risk of heart attack by 44 per cent.

And this was no small study either; a whopping 22,071 men took part in this research and were studied for five years.

67

Be in 'Flow'

A professor in Chicago has dedicated the last ten years of his life to studying what makes people happy, and his conclusion is that happiness is caused by a state called 'Flow'.

Mihalyi Cziksentmilhalyi describes this state as the halfway point between being relaxed and being stressed – in other words, he says we are happiest when filling our lives with challenging, involving activities that we do well.

As many gerontologists believe that those who are happiest tend to live longest, ask yourself, 'Do I have enough challenging, enjoyable activities in my life?'.

68

Eat your onions

Chinese researchers believe they've discovered a connection between low cancer rates and the consumption of onion and garlic, from the allium family of vegetables.

In an extensive research study, those people who reported eating the greatest number of allium vegetables had the fewest cases of cancer of the stomach.

Prevention magazine also reported a study conducted at Harvard University where doctors placed onion extract in a test tube with cancer cells and the cancer cell growth greatly slowed!

69

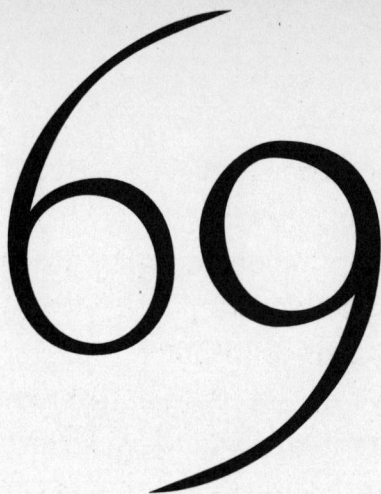

Have a regular Pap test

Most women over 65 don't have regular Pap tests, and many have never had one.

Yet the Australian Cancer Council recommends a test every two years, even if they've all been clear before.

The brilliant longevity book *Lifespan Plus* reports that the five-year survival rate for uterine cancer (which a Pap test can detect) is over 85 per cent when it's caught and treated early.

70

Watch out for the wok!

Food cooked in a Chinese wok may taste yummy, but the smoky fumes emanating from woks may lead to cancer, at least according to a study of Chinese women using oils in wok cooking.

The fact is that Chinese wok cooks have the same lung cancer rate as American women, yet they smoke only half as much. This is leading researchers to believe it may be the wok that's the culprit.

If you must use a wok, keep the kitchen well ventilated and keep the oil temperature down.

71

Drink in moderation

Don't kid yourself, alcohol can be a deadly killer.

In a study of over 106,000 Californians, scientists found that people who consumed more than three alcoholic drinks a day had triple the risk of developing rectal cancer than people who never drank.

Many other studies support these findings. So play it safe, and drink only occasionally and moderately.

72

Inspect your body regularly

Cancer of the testes can be spotted early by checking each testicle for any lumps.

Breast cancer can be detected by examining your breasts with your hands in an up and down rectangular pattern (it's more effective than the traditional concentric circle inspection technique).

Colorectal cancer can be checked by giving a stool sample once a year to your doctor.

These checks are quick, painless and could definitely save your life.

73

Peel your fruit and vegies

Beware of pesticides!

Fruits and vegetables often have pesticides on their skin, even after you've washed them.

The Natural Resources Defence Council reported a study showing that trimming celery reduced residues of methomyl (an insecticide believed to cause cancer) by 50 to 90 per cent.

Removing the outer leaves of lettuce will also reduce pesticide levels.

74

Keep noise levels down

A Japanese study revealed that people regularly exposed to noise were twice as likely to have high blood pressure than those in a quieter environment.

Vacuum cleaners, drills, loud music, and noisy traffic are all enough to lift blood pressure rates.

Either move to a quieter neighbourhood, or get yourself a good set of ear plugs!

Also, a 1998 Australian study showed that people who often listen to loud music through headphones could have major hearing problems in later life.

75

Take planes for long trips

Part of your living to 100 strategy should be to minimise the risk of fatal accidents.

So if you need to travel interstate, take a plane or train instead of driving. Although some people are scared of flying, statistically planes are much safer than cars, as are trains.

Amongst planes, the safest by far are those run by commuter airlines, followed by commercial charters then private planes.

76

Try Deprenyl

Mainly used as a drug for treating Parkinson's disease, Deprenyl (or Elderpryl) is fast becoming praised as an anti-aging pill.

Available by prescription only, and taken in small, professionally authorised doses, Deprenyl has been shown to help slow the aging process in male rats.

Studies have shown not only increased longevity in rats treated with Deprenyl, but also improved sexual activity and increased learning ability.

77

Watch out for gene medicine

Within years, the Human Genome Project will be completed; that is, the entire human gene pool will have been mapped and sequenced.

As a result, medical procedures to destroy and replace defective genes will become common.

Indeed, according to aging expert Professor Steven N Austad there are already over 100 clinical trials of gene based therapy underway. Keep an eye out for them. Many people predict they are the future of anti-aging medicine.

78

Try estrogen

For women, it's hard to find a better anti-aging medicine. Results from a variety of significant research studies indicate the following possible benefits for estrogen takers:

- increased longevity;
- reduced cholesterol;
- stronger bones;
- reduced risk of heart disease.

It's critical, however, that estrogen use be regularly monitored (blood, urine and saliva tests should be done three times annually) and that the medicine be taken consistently.

Also, ask your doctor whether your estrogen should be supplemented with progesterone.

79

Don't smoke dope

Many people believe marijuana is less dangerous than tobacco. Actually, the opposite is true. Marijuana is in fact more carcinogenic than tobacco, especially as a cause of throat cancer.

Dope is also harder on the lungs, as marijuana smokers typically inhale the smoke deeply and hold it inside them.

Finally, according to Professors Talalaj and Talalaj (father and son longevity experts), marijuana use leads to increased risk of mental illness such as schizophrenia. They also indicate that Ecstasy is a highly dangerous drug for the user's brain.

80

Wear sunglasses

Your eyes are vulnerable to ultraviolet (UV) rays. Those of us who don't wear sunglasses to protect against harmful UV rays are at risk of cancer of the eye.

Choose your glasses carefully though. Over 40 per cent of sunglasses actually can't filter out UV rays. So buy from an optometrist or get their recommendations on the most protective brands.

81

Beware of slimming remedies

Anything extreme is unlikely to be good for the body, but particularly keep an eye out for any slimming products containing Germander.

Although only a few years ago Germander was hugely popular (in France especially) as a slimming remedy, it was found to have serious side effects. These effects included severe liver poisoning.

Beware also of two Oriental herbs used occasionally in slimming products – *Stephania tetrandra* and *Magnolio officinalis* – both of which can lead to kidney problems.

82

Stay away from
artificial sweeteners

Many artificial sweeteners are made from cyclamates. While there is no conclusive research as to their effect on humans, there have been studies showing that animals fed with cyclamate suffered higher rates of bladder cancer. So perhaps it's best to avoid this substance.

Some other sweeteners have saccharin in them, and some studies have identified a link between the consumption of saccharin and bladder cancer.

That's why I stay away from these substances (which often appear in diet drinks and low-joule canned fruits). After all, better to be safe than sorry.

83

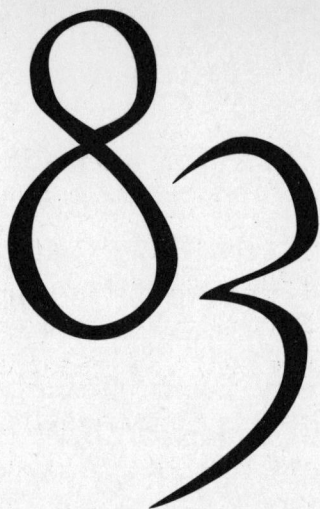

Check
electromagnetic fields

Power lines and electrical appliances could be highly injurious to you and your family's health. According to a leaked report from the National Council on Radiation Protection, a powerful body of impressive evidence now exists which suggests that very low exposure to EMFs (electromagnetic fields) can have long term harmful effects.

Various studies show that exposure to electromagnetic fields can lead to increased levels of leukaemia, Alzheimer's and decreased immune system efficiency.

So don't live near power lines and keep your use of electrical appliances to a minimum.

84

Apple juice can be dangerous!

A 1993 study by the Food and Drug Administration in the US found that around 25 per cent of apple juice tested had high levels of the toxin known as patulin. (It is suspected that the apple juices containing high levels of patulin were made from partially mouldy apples.)

It's not good news if the same is true in Australia, as evidence suggests patulin may suppress your immune system.

So please make sure your apple juice is made from only fresh apples.

85

Take smart drugs

One of the most exciting areas of medicine is that of brain enhancing drugs, or nootropics.

For example in Germany, nootropics are widely prescribed by doctors for slight memory disturbances and general brain boosting.

Let's consider Piracetam. A recent French study testing Piracetam produced dramatic results. Grenoble University Hospital gave 135 people varying doses of Piracetam. After six weeks, those given a higher dosage top scored on memory tests, even though prior to the study they had the lowest scores.

If Piracetam is not available in your country ask your physician about Deprenyl, Clonidine or Acetyl-l-carnitine.

86

The magic of
sleeping potions

As good sleep patterns are crucial to longevity, it's worth doing whatever you can to encourage a quality snooze.

One herb which has been well researched as an aid to sleep is Valerian root. (There are over 150 drugs made from Valerian root in Germany alone.) Valerian has been found to reduce the time it takes to get to sleep. (A good dosage is one teaspoon in warm water before bedtime.)

Other sleep potions include Kava Kava and GABA (Gamma-aminobutyric acid).

Don't forget the other tried and true sleep aids – chamomile and lemon balm tea, and lavender oil in a warm bath.

87

The Morning Power Questions

Being in a happy mood usually leads to less stress on your body and mind, even creating endorphins, or 'feel good' drugs, inside your brain.

But how do you get happy?

One method practised by self-development wunderkind Anthony Robbins is the Morning Power Questions.

By asking yourself the following questions each morning, and really thinking about the answers, we become more conscious of how lucky we are and our mood tends to improve.

1. What am I excited about in life right now (or what could I be excited about)?
2. What am I happy about in my life?
3. What am I enjoying in my life right now?
4. What am I grateful for in my life right now?
5. Who do I love and who loves me, and how does that make me feel?

88

Don't have much for dinner

As lean people tend to live longer than fat people, it's important to know how to encourage calorie burning.

One of the best tricks is to keep your evening meal small.

Studies indicate that those who eat most of their calories at breakfast and lunch lose more weight than people who eat the same amount, but late at night.

That's because food eaten earlier in the day is more likely to be burned off by the day's activities than an evening meal, which gets digested while you're asleep.

89

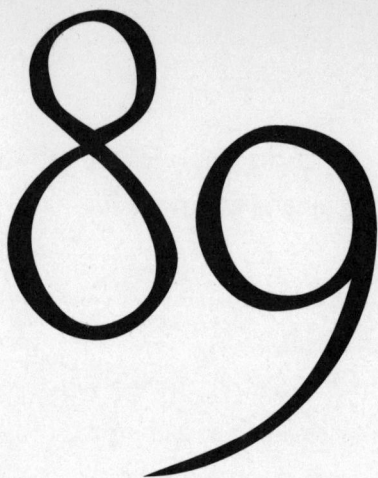

Know the facts of cancer

Cancer is a lot more preventable than most people imagine. Indeed, *Prevention* magazine quotes research estimating that fully 68 per cent of cancer could have been prevented.

Scientists say that 35 per cent of all cancer deaths are caused by bad diet, 30 per cent by regular smoking, 2 per cent by environmental pollution and 1 per cent by food additives.

Cancers that are particularly preventable include breast, bladder, liver, lung, larynx, skin, esophagus and stomach cancer.

Much of our immunity to cancer depends on what we eat, drink and breathe and, of course, our mental state.

90

Find the best doctor

If you're diagnosed with a serious disease the first thing to do is not panic.

The second is to become an expert on that disease, and the best doctors in the world to cure it.

You'd be amazed, for instance, at the different success rates some cancer specialists have – choose the right one and you can sometimes triple your chances of cure.

So be sure to check relevant alternative medicine sites on the Internet and search out the finest books on your particular disease.

For instance, one of the best books for cancer sufferers is *The Definitive Guide to Cancer* by Burton Goldberg, available in the United States or through Amazon.com books on the Net (www.amazon.com).

91

Stretch it

Lots of people exercise, but not so many work on their flexibility.

That's a big mistake, because daily stretching exercises can be a huge benefit to your body, especially as you get older.

According to Dr John Bland, author of the intriguingly titled book *Live Long Die Fast*, stretching exercises will bring more nutrients to the muscles, prevent injuries, increase range of motion, improve body shape, reduce muscle tension and pain, help co-ordination and much more.

See your local gym instructor for the best methods, or book an hour with a personal trainer to create a regimen especially suited for you.

92

Pray

According to the eminent researcher Dr Herbert Benson, research on the faithful indicates that those who regularly pray have lower cholesterol, lower stress and significantly less risk of heart attack than those who don't. The results also indicate that these people have a higher level of happiness than the typical atheist.

Another research study available from The John Templeton Foundation showed that religious people had reduced depression and anger, and were generally better able to cope with the troubles of life than non-religious people.

93

Walking works

Is walking the king of exercises?

A lot of doctors think so.

After all, vigorous walking provides many of the benefits of running and aerobics, without the intensity and muscle stress of these training methods.

And because you can exercise for longer when you walk, your metabolism stays higher longer, leading to excellent weight loss results.

Even people with serious ailments can benefit from walking. It's great medicine for those with lung disease, arthritis, osteoporosis and hardening of the arteries.

The other good thing about walking is that you can do it even in your nineties, and still get enormous benefits from it . . .

94

Fall in love

We all know love makes the world go round. Well, it may also keep you going around, at least for a few years longer.

Scientists have found that people in love tend to produce more age-reducing hormones such as estrogen, progesterone, DHEA and Human Growth Hormone than people who aren't.

Because they're usually happier, couples in love also often have an immune system that is stronger than normal.

Finally, those in love are also usually less stressed. It seems that work and social troubles are far less of a burden when you're floating on Cloud 9.

However, romance can be a two-edged sword, and if things turn sour and your love life becomes misery, the exact opposite physiological changes can occur – until the unlucky lover recovers or finds a new special partner.

95

Visualise being young

Long used by Olympic athletes to maximise performance, visualisation can actually keep you younger, longer.

Here's how it works.

Over 80 per cent of your brain is categorised as the subconscious mind. Researchers have found that the subconscious accepts any information given to it, regardless of whether it is true or not.

So by visualising yourself each day as being young and vibrant, you will soon believe you are. And when you believe it, you'll start behaving like it.

If this seems a little far-fetched, be aware that there has been over 30 years of research on visualisation with some outstanding results. It definitely works. The key is to be consistent with your visualisation, picturing yourself young and healthy for at least five minutes every day.

96

Think positively about aging

You'll age better if you feel better about aging.

That's easy to say, but harder to do. There are so many myths about how the quality of life crumbles with old age that many people are terrified of it.

To help dispel these fears, here are some aging facts:

- People over 65 get fewer illnesses than young people!
- Your brain can not only remain agile, but actually improve, even in your nineties.
- A full one-third of people over 65 either report that these are their best years ever, or that they expect the best is still to come.

So relax, and stay positive about the wonderful journey ahead of you!

97

Help people

In 1982 a nation-wide study was done in China on the many centenarians in that country. The researchers attempted to discover the common lifestyle characteristics of their longest living citizens.

One of their surprising discoveries was that many of China's 100-year-olds were deeply involved in helping people, often for no money, and placed contribution to their neighbours as a high daily priority.

98

Eat less

Tests on a wide variety of warm-blooded animals prove that restricting the total amount of food increases longevity.

Experts believe less food leads to less fat, less poisons and less stress on the digestive system.

So go easy at meal time, and you'll enjoy many more meals to come . . .

99

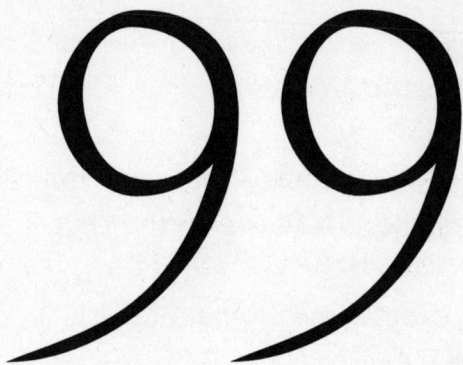

Enjoy a regular massage

Adored by everyone, young or old, a good massage is also a highly effective way to stay healthy.

When correctly administered, massage techniques help reduce the build up of lactic acid in the muscles, invigorate internal organs and gently stimulate blood flow.

Massage is also an extraordinarily effective antidote to stress, a well-established life shortener.

Major styles of massage include Swedish, Chinese and Western remedial.

100

Become an anti-aging expert

Albert Einstein once said that you could become a world renowned expert in any field just by reading an hour a day for life.

So why not become an expert on longevity? It will open up an amazing new world for you.

There's so much research available to dig into. As well as hundreds of books on the subject, there's a biannual conference of the American Academy of Anti-aging Medicine, numerous anti-aging journals and scores of longevity web-sites on the Internet. It really is a fascinating world.

It's also a great way to make sure your last 50 years of life are every bit as great as your first!

There are new titles coming out all the time, but here is my current Top Ten list of longevity books. Be sure to check them out.

Appendix

1. *Stopping the Clock* by Doctors Klatz and Goldman (Keats Publishing)

2. *Dare to Be 100* by Walter M Bortz II MD (Fireside)

3. *Feel 30 for the Next 50 Years* by David W Johnson PhD (Avon Books)

4. *Look Ten Years Younger, Live Ten Years Longer* by David Ryback (Prentice Hall)

5. *Quantum Longevity* by Dr Vincent Giampapa – available from Longevity Institute International in New Jersey, USA

If you would like to find out more about how anti-aging therapies can help keep you young and healthy, contact the Redwood Anti-Aging Clinic on 1800 080 880.

Siimon Reynolds
When They Zig You Zag

In this breakthrough book, advertising ace and best-selling motivational author Siimon Reynolds shows you how to transform every aspect of your life and achieve your dreams by creating your own path, instead of following the paths of others.

When They Zig You Zag will show you how to achieve your goals faster, stay relaxed, balance your life, maximise your brain power, and experience more joy in life. It is a must-read for anyone looking to squeeze the most out of their life and achieve spectacular levels of success.

Siimon Reynolds
Become Happy in Eight Minutes

This is *not* hype. These are *not* mind games. Use these techniques properly and it is physiologically impossible not to get into a better mood. They are based on decades of research on how the brain works. They'll work for the young, they'll work for the old. You truly are only ever eight minutes away from feeling happy.

Isn't that a lovely thought?